YOU CAN
SHUN ALCOHOLISM:
Escape Route From The Addiction Called
" *Alcoholism* "
Kelvin K. Walker

Table of Content

PREFACE

Alcohol is a central nervous system depressant. This means that it's a medicine that slows down brain exertion. It can change your mood, gesture, and tone- control. It can beget problems with memory and allow easy. Alcohol can also affect your collaboration and physical control. Alcohol also has effects on the other organs in your body. For illustration, it can raise your blood pressure and heart rate.

However, it could make you throw up If you drink too much. Alcohol's goods vary from person to person, depending on a variety of factors, including How much you drank, how snappily you drank it, the quantity of food you ate before drinking, your age, your sex, your ethnicity, your physical condition, whether or not you have a family history of alcohol problems. Moderate drinking for women is no further than one standard drink a day. For most men, moderate drinking is no further than two standard drinks a day. Indeed though moderate drinking may be safe for numerous people, there are still pitfalls. Moderate drinking can raise the threat of death from certain cancers and heart conditions.

In the United States, a standard drink contains about 14 grams of pure alcohol, which is set up in ounces of beer(5 alcohol content) 5 ounces of wine(12 alcohol content) ounces or a" shot" of distilled spirits or liquor(40 alcohol content) Some people shouldn't drink alcohol at each, including those who Are recovering from an alcohol use complaint(AUD) or are unfit to control the quantum they drink, are under age 21, are pregnant or trying to come pregnant, are taking drugs that can interact with alcohol, have medical conditions that get can worse if you drink alcohol, are planning on driving, and people about to operate a ministry. Inappropriate drinking includes binge drinking and heavy alcohol use Binge drinking is drinking so much as formerly that your blood alcohol attention(BAC) position is 0.08 or further.

For a man, this generally happens after having 5 or further drinks within many hours. For a woman, it's after about 4 or more drinks within many hours. Heavy alcohol use is having further than 4 drinks on any day for men or further than 3 drinks for women Binge drinking raises your threat of injuries, auto crashes, and alcohol poisoning. It also puts you off getting violent or being the victim of violence.

Heavy alcohol use over a long period may beget health problems similar to Alcohol use complaints, Liver conditions, including cirrhosis and adipose liver complaint, Heart conditions, Increased threat of certain cancers, and Increased threat of injuries. Heavy alcohol use can also beget problems at home, at work, and with musketeers. But treatment can help.

Chapter 1: The Concept of Alcoholism

Alcoholism is the most severe form of alcohol abuse and involves the incapability to manage drinking habits. It also generally pertains to an alcohol use complaint. Inordinate alcohol use can damage all organ systems, but it particularly affects the brain, heart, liver, pancreas, and vulnerable systems. Alcoholism can affect internal illness, distraction Tremens, Wernicke – Korsakoff pattern, irregular twinkle, a disabled vulnerable response, liver cirrhosis, and increased cancer threat.

Drinking during gestation can affect fetal alcohol diapason disorders. Women are generally more sensitive than men to the dangerous goods of alcohol, primarily due to their lower body weight, lower capacity to metabolize alcohol, and advanced proportion of body fat.

In a small number of individuals, severe alcohol abuse eventually leads to cognitive impairment and foursquare madness. Individuals floundering with drunkenness frequently feel as though they can not serve typically without alcohol. This can lead to a wide range of issues and impact professional pretensions, particular matters, connections, and overall health. Over time, the serious side goods of harmonious alcohol abuse can worsen and produce dangerous complications. The warning signs of alcohol abuse are veritably conspicuous. Other times, they can take longer to surface. When alcohol dependence is discovered in its early stages, the chance for a successful recovery increases significantly.

Common signs of alcoholism include; Being unfit to control alcohol consumption, pining for alcohol when you're not drinking, Putting alcohol above particular liabilities, Feeling the need to keep drinking further, Spending a substantial quantum of plutocrats on alcohol, and carrying else after drinking. However, it's important to find treatment options that will help you protest your alcohol dependence to check If you feel as though your alcohol consumption is taking a risk on your life. Your croaker will be suitable to offer professional medical backing if you're concerned about your drinking. Seeking help for drunkenness sooner rather than later gets you back on track to living a healthy, fulfilling life.

Stages of Alcoholism

Alcohol use complaints are grouped into four stages; Pre-Alcoholic Stage, Early- Stage Alcoholism(Prodromal), Middle Alcoholic Phase, and End-Stage Alcoholism. Each stage has colorful symptoms and can beget dangerous side effects. However, any type of alcohol abuse can spiral out of control, If left undressed.

Pre-Alcoholic Stage

The pre-alcoholic stage occurs before alcohol is ever a real problem. It's delicate to identify because alcohol has yet to beget any problems and drinking has not come obsessive. Indeed those in the pre-alcoholic stage are doubtful to fete that their drinking may ultimately progress into a commodity serious. The way alcohol interacts with the body and mind is complex. It mimics certain chemicals, GABA and glutamate, that the brain naturally produces and are needed for proper functioning. The former causes people to relax while the ultimate is excitatory and makes them more active. The further a person drinks, the further their body becomes dependent on ethanol to release these neurotransmitters rather than releasing them naturally. This is how physical alcohol dependence develops.

The pre-alcoholic stage is constructive; people go in one of two directions. Those who begin using alcohol as a tool someone uses to decompress after a long day, bolster themselves in social situations, or help them fall asleep progress into the coming stage of drunkenness. Those who find druthers to drinking either stay in the pre-alcoholic stage or move down from drinking altogether.

How to identify an existent in the Pre-Alcoholic Stage

It's frequently delicate to determine whether someone is in the pre-alcoholic stage. Their drinking hasn't veered far from regular social drinking. People in the pre-alcoholic stage may enjoy drinking more constantly than those around them but it isn't overtly conspicuous in most people. These drinkers have a drink in their hand at most or all social gatherings. You might notice it if they use it as their go-to way to decompress after a grueling day or long week.

However, they can't bear to face a social gathering without a drink, or need alcohol to relax, If they regularly calculate on alcohol as a managing medium. Seeking treatment during the pre-alcoholic stage is possible but is largely doubtful. Signs of the pre-alcoholic stage counting on alcohol to decompress or relax demanding a drink to engage in social situations Using alcohol to manage uncomfortable passions or feelings.

Early- Stage Alcoholism(Prodromal)

Early- stage Alcoholism, or the prodromal phase, is when people begin binge drinking regularly and may indeed black out sometimes. This behavior may be a sign of trial with alcohol gone too far, especially in the case of adolescents or youthful adults. However, they keep drinking past a certain point, If their drinking continues. Binge drinking is characterized by the consumption of around four drinks within two hours for women and five drinks within two hours for men.

However, it's time for them to seriously review their drinking habits If this is a normal quantum for their loved ones. Enjoying the sensation of rapid-fire onset drunkenness and drinking to seek intoxication as snappily as possible is dangerous and may indicate a deeper problem. individualities in this stage may not be drinking every day or indeed every week. They still use alcohol constantly and can't imagine a " good night out " without it. They drink heavily under the guise of " having a good time with musketeers " or " relaxing after a long week at the office. " Anyhow of their logic, however, regularly drinking to redundant flowers the mind and body for the development of a more serious problem with alcohol latterly on. relating to individualities in Early- Stage Alcoholism.

Early- stage Alcoholism Is easier to notice than the pre-alcoholism stage. Your friend or family member in early-stage drunkenness will regularly binge drink or drink to the point of bartering out. They'll likely joke about their knockouts or mention they won't drink that much again. Still, they'll inescapably drink that much again not long later. Over time it becomes a cycle of binge drinking, bartering out, swearing to cut back, and also starting again. Still, you have a right to be concerned, If you notice they continue drinking heavily and bartering out.

Keep an eye on their drinking actions to see whether they progress further. Indeed if they never progress past this stage, regular binge drinking isn't a healthy way to consume alcohol. Signs of early-stage drunkenness Regular binge drinking " Bartering out "(memory loss caused by drinking) Difficulties controlling the quantum they drink Swearing they'll cut back or stop but having trouble doing so.

Middle Alcoholic Phase

During this stage, your condition may come apparent to musketeers and family, although some people can come largely complete at hiding their problem drinking. One of the main issues with this complaint is how easy it becomes to lie to yourself as well. However, you'll frequently play down the amount you drink and find ways of explaining the behavior If you're in this phase.

You may start to witness consequences at work or the academy due to your habit and find yourself regularly hungover and pining for more alcohol. Signs similar to drinking at work, while looking after children or when driving are pointers of this stage. You've likely come more perverse, and alcohol may start to affect you else. You'll need to drink further to achieve the same goods you used to feel and frequently pass out from alcohol. Changes in your body similar to facial greenishness, stomach bloating, shaking, sweating and memory setbacks start to affect you. Relating Someone with Middle-Stage Alcoholism The farther someone's drinking progresses, the easier it becomes to notice their lack of control. Middle-stage drunkenness is when their drinking problem reaches more serious situations.

Clear examples of progressive alcoholism include; placing drinking ahead of their family, their job, or their education. Treatment is most salutary for those at the point of middle-stage drunkenness. They've reached a place where their health declined too far and they can make some extreme changes in their lives. Attending alcohol recovery at this stage will be incredibly salutary.

End-Stage Alcoholism

In this phase, the goods of long-term alcohol abuse will start to come apparent. You might have tried and failed to stop or cut down on drinking several times, too. Alcohol consumption becomes an each-day affair, and your precedences change to grease drinking as the most important aspect of your life. However, the sadness and solicitude associated with these life events could make the situation worse, If you've lost your job or you're in fiscal trouble.

End- stage Alcoholism is the most serious point to reach. It's apparent when someone is at the end stages of their alcohol dependence. They see severe impacts on their health, connections, employment, finances, and overall satisfaction with life. Paranoia is constantly seen during this phase. Some people — known as performing rummies — can still maintain their life during this phase, but this is rare and likely to lead to liver damage or other alcohol-related illnesses. However, don't continue down this dangerous path, If you feel like your drinking problem is habitual but your life isn't falling piecemeal. This complaint is progressive, and your health will ultimately bear the mass.

Chapter 2: Why People Drink

There are colorful reasons why people start drinking, some of the most common is to;

Relieve Stress

Counting on alcohol to reduce diurnal life stressors can impact the liability of developing drunkenness. Since alcohol is a depressant and an opiate, drinking produces passion of pleasure. Still, frequent drinking builds forbearance, taking you to consume further alcohol to achieve the same effects.

Feel Good

Consuming alcohol can give some people a break from reality. It offers a sense of relief from underpinning issues your mind may be trying to escape from. Still, continual alcohol use to get through the day or week can turn into a serious drinking problem.

Manage With Loss

Losing a family member or friend can take a risk on you emotionally, physically, and mentally. Alcohol can ease the grief you're feeling and is used to get through delicate times. Depending on alcohol, indeed temporarily, can be helical in a drinking problem.

Overcome Anxiety

Some people are naturally anxious, causing them to constantly worry. Drinking lowers an existent's inhibitions and makes them more comfortable in social situations. Over time, however, this can lead to addicting actions.

Lack Of Connection

Numerous people drink because they don't feel adequately connected to others. They believe that alcohol will either fill the void or conceivably make it easier for them to forge new bonds. Still, the contrary generally ends up being true.

Shame

Shame is one of the most delicate feelings for numerous to manage, and it's also one of the most traumatic. While alcohol can temporarily mask shame with false passions, it also causes numerous individuals to engage in reckless or foolish actions that can later beget them to feel indeed lesser shame, which can beget a downcast curl.

Trauma

Treatment professionals see some type of trauma in nearly every case that they treat. There are numerous forms of trauma, but they're each painful events that take a risk on the internal health of the person floundering with dependence. For numerous, treating undetermined trauma is the key to their recovery.

Drinking too much on a single occasion or long-term can take a serious risk to your health. Some effects of alcohol may have a minor effect on your health, while others can be severe or life-changing.

Chapter 3: The Myths of Alcohol

Myth 1: You have to respect a person who can hold his/ her liquor. The person who can drink large amounts of alcohol without feeling the" normal" goods may have developed a forbearance to alcohol. Forbearance comes from the habitual use of alcohol that results in physical and internal adaptation to its presence in the body. The development of forbearance is shown by an increase in the quantum of alcohol needed to produce the asked goods and can indicate the onset of physical dependence.

Myth 2: Alcohol can be used as a food supplement. Alcohol has no nutritive value. It contains no vitamins, minerals, or proteins. It does contain a significant number of calories, still. The calories can produce an immediate source of energy which causes food that's typically used for energy products to be changed into fat and stored in the body for after-use.

Myth 3: Alcohol warms the body. The direct action of alcohol causes a drop in the internal body temperature in the ensuing process. The blood vessels are opened(dilated) on the skin shells and the blood is cooled by lesser exposure to the external terrain. As the cooled blood circulates, the core temperature is lowered gradationally, but significantly. This process is continued as long as alcohol is present in the body.

Myth 4: Alcohol is a stimulant medicine. Alcohol is a depressant; it sedates the central nervous system. One of the first areas of the brain to be affected is the cerebral cortex, which controls judgment, tone-control, and inhibitions. The depression on this part of the brain may affect hyperexcitable behavior, as inhibitions are lost.

Myth 5: Hangovers are caused by switching drinks. Hangovers are caused by the quantity of alcohol consumed and the rate at which it's consumed, not by the kind of alcohol consumed. While metabolizing alcohol, the liver can not perform its normal functions, one of which is keeping the blood sugar at normal attention. The result of this state is called hypoglycemia, or lower-than-normal blood sugar. The change in blood vessels can beget headaches. Incipiently, a leftover is a"mini-withdrawal." When the central nervous system is released from the depressed state, the contrary state develops- feeling edgy and perverse. This effect is known as the" answer."

Myth 6: Alcoholics drink every day. Alcoholics are of numerous kinds: those who drink daily, those who drink on weekends, those who drink on binges which could do weeks, months, or indeed times piecemeal. The measure of drunkenness isn't when or how frequently one drinks, but whether or not one can control the drinking once it begins.

Myth 7: You can not become an alcoholic by drinking only beer. Americans drink nearly ten times as important beer as they do" hard" liquor. Although the content of alcohol in beer is fairly low, this means that one-half the alcohol drunk is consumed as beer. Given these data, it seems reasonable to say that numerous alcoholics are only beer alkies.

Myth 8: Black coffee or a cold shower sobers a drunk. Black coffee and cold showers only produce wide-awake drunks. Only time will relieve the body of alcohol. There's no given way of speeding the metabolic process of barring alcohol from the body.

Myth 9: I can drink and still be in control. Drinking impairs your judgment, which increases the liability that you'll make a commodity you will later lament. It increases the chance that you'll beget detriment to others and/ or not be apprehensive of implicit troubles around you. Critical decision-making capacities are formerly lowered long before a person shows physical signs of intoxication.

Myth 10: Drinking isn't all those dangerous many pitfalls are associated with drinking, including disabled driving, unintentional injuries, violence, unsafe sexual behavior self-murder attempts, overdoses, and death. Indeed council scholars who do not drink may witness secondary goods, similar to disrupted study and sleep, or be involved in an alcohol-related assault.

Myth 11: It's okay to drink to keep up with guys, women process alcohol else. No matter how much joe drinks, if you drink the same quantity as your manly musketeers your blood alcohol attention will tend to be advanced, putting you at a lesser threat for detriment.

Myth 12: I can manage to drive well enough after many drinksThe goods of alcohol start sooner than people realize, with mild impairment(up to0.05 blood alcohol attention(BAC)) starting to affect speech, memory, attention, collaboration, and balance. And if you're under 21, driving after drinking any quantum of alcohol is illegal and you could lose your license. The pitfalls of a fatal crash for motorists with positive BAC compared with other motorists increase as the BAC increases, and the pitfalls increase further acutely for motorists younger than age 21 than for aged motorists. Critical decision-making capacities and driving-affiliated chops are formerly lowered long before a person shows physical signs of intoxication.

Myth 13: I Am Too Old to Have a Drinking Problem has been expanded. You may suppose that drinking problems have to start beforehand in life. Some people develop problems with drinking at an age. One reason is that people become more sensitive to alcohol as they get older. Or they may take drugs that make the goods of alcohol stronger. Some aged grown-ups may start to drink further because they're tired or feel lonely or depressed.

Indeed if you've never drank that much when you were youthful, you can have problems with drinking as you get older. What's a healthy range of drinking for men and women over 65 times? Experts recommend no further than 3 drinks in a single day or no further than an aggregate of 7 drinks a week. A drink is defined as 12 fluid ounces(355 mL) of beer, 5 fluid ounces(148 mL) of wine, or 1 ½ fluid ounces(45 mL) of liquor.

Chapter 4: The Effects of Alcoholism

The effect of alcohol is grouped into short-term effects of alcohol and long-term effects of alcohol.

Short-Term Effects of Alcohol

Temporary effects you might notice while drinking alcohol(or shortly later) can include passions of relaxation or dizziness, a sense of swoon or giddiness, mood changes, lowered inhibitions, impulsive gestures, braked or vocalized speech, nausea, and vomiting, diarrhea, headache, changes in hail, vision, and perception, loss of collaboration, trouble fastening or making opinions, loss of knowledge or gaps in memory(frequently called a knockout).
Some of these effects, like a relaxed mood or lowered inhibitions, might show up snappily after just one drink. Others, like loss of knowledge or vocalized speech, may develop after many drinks. Dehumidification-related effects, like nausea, headache, and dizziness, might not appear for many hours, and they can also depend on what you drink, how important you drink, and if you also drink water.
These effects might not last veritably long, but that doesn't make them insignificant. freakishness, loss of collaboration, and mood changes can affect your judgment and behavior and contribute to further far-reaching goods, including accidents, injuries, and opinions you later lament.

Long-Term Effects of Alcohol

Alcohol use can also lead to further continuing enterprises that extend beyond your mood and health. Some long-term effects of constantly drinking alcohol can include patient changes in mood, including anxiety and perversity, wakefulness and other sleep enterprises, a weakened vulnerable system(meaning you might get sick more frequently), changes in libido and sexual function, changes in appetite and weight, problems with memory and attention, difficulty fastening on tasks, increased pressure and conflict in romantic and family connections.

Alcohol's physical effects on the body

Here's a breakdown of alcohol's effects on your internal organs and body processes.

Digestive and endocrine glands

The connection between alcohol consumption and your digestive system might not feel incontinently clear. The side effects frequently only appear after the damage has happened. Continuing to drink can worsen these symptoms. Drinking can damage the tissues in your digestive tract, precluding your bowel from digesting food and absorbing nutrients and vitamins duly.

In time, this damage can beget malnutrition. Heavy drinking can also lead to gas bloating, a feeling of wholeness in your tummy, diarrhea or painful droppings, ulcers, or hemorrhoids(due to dehumidification and constipation). Ulcers can beget dangerous internal bleeding, which can occasionally be fatal without prompt opinion and treatment.

Drinking too much alcohol over time may cause inflammation of the pancreas, performing in pancreatitis. Pancreatitis can spark the release of pancreatic digestive enzymes and beget abdominal pain.

Seditious damage

Your liver helps break down and remove poisons and dangerous substances(including alcohol) from your body. Long-term alcohol use interferes with this process. It also increases your threat of alcohol-related liver complaints and habitual liver inflammation. An alcohol-related liver complaint is a potentially life-changing condition that leads to poisons and waste buildup in your body. habitual liver inflammation can beget scarring or cirrhosis. When scar towel forms, it may permanently damage your liver.

Sugar situations

The pancreas helps regulate how your body uses insulin and responds to glucose. However, you could witness low blood sugar, or hypoglycemia, If your pancreas and liver don't function duly due to pancreatitis or liver complaint. A damaged pancreas can also help your body from producing enough insulin to use sugar. This can lead to hyperglycemia or too important sugar in the blood. However, you may witness lesser complications and side goods related to diabetes, If your body can't manage and balance your blood sugar situations. Avoid inordinate quantities of alcohol if you have diabetes or hypoglycemia.

Central nervous system

One major way to recognize alcohol's impact on your body? Understanding how it affects your central nervous system. Vocalized speech, a crucial sign of intoxication, happens because alcohol reduces communication between your brain and body. This makes speech and collaboration think response time and balance more delicate. That's one major reason why you should not drive after drinking.

Over time, alcohol can damage your central nervous system. You might notice impassiveness and chinking in your bases and hands. Drinking can also affect your capability to produce long-term recollections, suppose easily, make rational choices, and regulate your feelings over time. Drinking can also damage your anterior lobe, the part of the brain responsible for administrative functions, like abstract logic, decision timber, social behavior, and performance. habitual heavy drinking can also beget endless brain damage, including the Wernicke- Korsakoff pattern, a brain complaint that affects memory.

Circulatory system

Habitual drinking can affect your heart and lungs, raising your threat of developing heart-related

health issues. Circulatory system complications include high blood pressure, irregular twinkle, difficulty pumping blood through the body, stroke, heart attack, heart complaint, heart failure, difficulty absorbing vitamins and minerals from food can beget fatigue, and anemia, a condition where you have low red blood cell count.

Sexual and reproductive health

Drinking alcohol can lower your inhibitions, so you might assume alcohol can ramp up your fun in the bedroom. In reality, however, heavy drinking can help coitus hormone product, lower your libido, keep you from getting or maintaining construction, and make it delicate to achieve orgasm, inordinate drinking may affect your menstrual cycle and potentially increase your threat for gravidity.

Cadaverous and muscle system

Long-term alcohol use can affect bone viscosity, leading to thinner bones and adding the threat of fractures if you fall. Weakened bones may also heal slower. Drinking alcohol can also lead to muscle weakness, cramping, and ultimately atrophy.

Immune system

Drinking heavily reduces your body's naturally vulnerable system. A weakened vulnerable system has a harder time guarding you against origins and contagions. People who drink heavily over a long period are also more likely to develop pneumonia or tuberculosis than the general population.

The World Health Organization(WHO) links about 8.1 percent of trusted sources of all tuberculosis cases worldwide to alcohol consumption. Drinking alcohol can also factor into your cancer threat Frequent drinking can increase your threat of developing mouth, throat, bone, esophagus, colon, or liver cancer. Drinking and using tobacco together can further increase your risk of developing mouth or throat cancer.

Chapter 5: Sure Ways to Curb Alcoholism

The probable ways to help check Alcoholism include;

Put it in writing: Making a list of the reasons to curtail your drinking such as feeling healthier, sleeping better, or perfecting your connections can motivate you.

Set a drinking thing: Set a limit on how much you'll drink. You should keep your drinking below the recommended guidelines of no further than one standard drink per day for women and men aged 65 and older, and no further than two standard drinks per day for men under 65. These limits may be too high for people who have certain medical conditions or for some aged grown-ups. Your croaker can help you determine what is right for you.

Keep a journal of your drinking: For three to four weeks keep track of every time you have a drink. Include information about what and how important you drank as well as where you were. Compare this to your goal. However, bandy it with your croaker or another health professional, If you are having trouble sticking to your thing.

Don't Keep Alcohol At Home: You can't drink it If you don't have alcohol at home. Being unfit to simply go to the cupboard or the fridge to snare a drink can keep you from developing a pattern of alcohol use that can fluently develop into abuse or dependence. Confining access to alcohol at home can also prevent drinking out of tedium or your feelings. Only drinking in social settings helps you maintain some responsibility as well.

Keep up your water and food input: If you're thirsty, reach for water or a non-alcohol volition rather than alcohol. And make sure to alternate your alcoholic drinks with non-alcoholic drinks. A glass of water, soda pop water, juice, or a soft drink will do the trick. Drinking on an empty stomach will increase the rate at which alcohol is metabolized in your body. Eating ahead or while you drink alcohol will help it be absorbed into the bloodstream at a lower rate.

Not minding how much food you eat or water you drink, our bodies only break down one standard drink of alcohol every hour, on average. So drinking a glass of water or having a plate of food after you've started drinking won't inescapably help reduce the effect alcohol has on our body or reduce our blood alcohol attention(BAC).

Know Your Drinking Limits: Frequently, people try to set their limits on alcohol consumption. Still, the limits of alcohol use and abuse are easily outlined by the National Institute on Alcohol Use and Alcoholism(NIAAA). Low-threat drinking for women means no further than seven drinks per week and no further than three in one day. For men, no further than 14 drinks per week, no further than four per day. The suggested quantity if a person chooses to drink is one per day for women and two for men. These recommendations aren't for people who formerly have an alcohol use complaint or have completed a substance use program. These recommendations may also vary for people with health problems or different body types.

There's frequently the argument that no one drinks that little; still, the NIAAA has set up that 35 percent of people don't drink at all, 37 percent always drink in low-threat situations, and only 28 percent are heavy alkies. Change your " after work routine " If you've gotten into the habit of reaching for a glass of wine or a beer after work to help de-stress, try changing up your routine by changing some healthier druthers.

For illustration, try changing an after-work exertion, similar as going for a walk or run or doing another form of exertion, get into another hobby horse that doesn't involve alcohol, or if you're keen for a drink, try putting the kettle on or reaching for a delicious non-alcohol volition.

Drink sluggishly: Belt your drink. Drink soda pop, water, or juice after having an alcoholic libation. Never drink on an empty stomach.

Choose alcohol-free days: Decide not to drink a day or two each week. You may want to hesitate for a week or a month to see how you feel physically and emotionally without alcohol in your life. Taking a break from alcohol can be a good way to start drinking lower.

Watch for peer pressure: Practice ways to say no politely. You don't have to drink just because others are, and you should not feel indebted to accept every drink you are offered. Stay down from people who encourage you to drink. There are people you can spend time with and places you can go where alcohol isn't the focal point. However, you'll also be less likely to drink, If you spend time with people who don't drink or don't drink frequently.

Keep busy: Take a walk, play sports, go out to eat, or catch a movie. When you are at home, pick up a new hobby horse or readdress an old one. oil, board games, playing a musical instrument, woodworking — these and other conditioning are great druthers to drinking.

Ask for support: Cutting down on your drinking may not always be easy. Let musketeers and family members know that you need their support. Your croaker, counselor, or therapist may also be suitable to offer help.

Guard against temptation: Steer clear of people and places that make you want to drink. However, similar to leaves or recesses, develop a plan for managing them in advance, If you associate drinking with certain events. Cover your passions. When you are upset, lonely, or angry, you may be tempted to reach for a drink. Try to cultivate new, healthy ways to manage stress.

Be patient: Most people who successfully cut down or stop drinking altogether do so only after several attempts. You will presumably have lapses, but do not let them keep you from reaching your long-term thing. There is no final endpoint, as the process generally requires ongoing trouble.

Think Positively: Keep away all passions of doom and gloom, there's no need to be frustrated just think how proud your family and friends will be proud of you when you get out of the addiction and most importantly how proud you will be when you get out of it.

Most of these probable ways such as looking out for peer pressure, asking for support, being apprehensive of temptation, and being patient can also be helpful for people who want to give up alcohol fully. Once you've cut back on your drinking(so you are at or below the recommended guidelines), examine your drinking habits regularly to see if you are maintaining this position of drinking.

Some people attain their thing only to find that old habits crop up again later. However, consult your croaker, If this happens., there's no need to be miserable. Just suppose how proud your family and musketeers will be of you when you get out of this dependence. Most importantly, suppose how proud you'll be when you get out of it. Some of these strategies similar to watching for peer pressure, keeping busy, asking for support, being apprehensive of temptation, and being patient can also be helpful for people who want to give up alcohol fully.

Once you've cut back on your drinking(so you are at or below the recommended guidelines), examine your drinking habits regularly to see if you are maintaining this position of drinking. Some people attain their thing only to find that old habits crop up again later. However, consult your croaker, If this happens.

Chapter 6: Treatment

Choosing to seek help for alcohol dependence is one of the biggest opinions you'll face. There are different forms of treatment available grounded on the frequency of alcohol consumption and inflexibility of alcohol abuse.

Recovering from alcohol dependence is a process that continues long after recovery. It takes commitment to practice and apply the ways you learn in recovery, comforting, support groups, and other types of therapy. Although treatment plans are generally personalized for each case, treatment generally follows a structure.

Detoxification: The first stage in alcohol dependence recovery is detoxification. This phase should be completed with the help of medical professionals due to the eventuality of serious, uncomfortable pullout symptoms. numerous times, individuals are given a drug to help palliate the painful side effects of a pullout.

Medication

Three medications are presently approved in the United States to help people stop or reduce their drinking and help relapse. They're specified by a primary care doctor or other health professional and may be used alone or in combination with counseling. This includes;

Antabuse(Disulfiram): Antabuse(disulfiram) was the first drug approved for the treatment of alcohol abuse and alcohol dependence. It works by causing a severe adverse response when someone taking the drug consumes alcohol. the utmost people who take it'll heave after a drink of alcohol. This, in turn, is allowed to produce interference with drinking.

Naltrexone: Naltrexone is sold under the brand names Revia and Depade. An extended-release, yearly injectable form of naltrexone is retailed under the trade name Vivitrol. It works in the brain by blocking the high that people witness when they drink alcohol or take opioids like heroin and cocaine. When combined with psychosocial remedy, naltrexone could reduce alcohol jones and drop relapse rates in rummies.

Campral(Acamprosate): Campral(acamprosate) is the most recent drug approved for the treatment of alcohol dependence or drunkenness in theU.S. It works by homogenizing alcohol-related changes in the brain, reducing some of the extended physical torture and emotional discomfort people can witness when they quit drinking(also known as the post-acute pullout pattern) that can lead to relapse.

For anyone allowing treatment, talking to a primary care croaker is an important first step; he or she can be a good source for treatment referrals and specifics. A primary care Doctor can also estimate a case's drinking pattern, help draft a treatment plan, estimate overall health, and assess if specifics for alcohol may be applicable.

Rehabilitation: There are two types of recuperation that help treat alcohol use disorder; inpatient rehabilitation and outpatient rehabilitation. Inpatient rehabs are ferocious treatment programs that bear you to check into an installation for a certain period, generally 30, 60, or 90 days. Outpatient recovery allows individuals to share in a recovery program while continuing with their diurnal life. Talk with your doctor about treatment options to choose the stylish form of recovery for you.

Maintenance: The recovery process doesn't end with the completion of recovery. Long-term sobriety requires ongoing remedy and may number of support groups, comforting, and other recovery coffers. These will make sure you maintain sobriety and continue on a happy, healthy path for months and times to come.

Behavioral Treatments: Behavioral treatments are aimed at changing drinking behavior through comforting. They're led by health professionals and supported by studies showing they can be beneficial. Psychotherapy is the classic approach to having a discussion. During psychotherapy, a case is addressed to a trained psychologist about their problems and behaviors. A talk therapy session could take place in a one-to-one, group, or family setting. A case and their psychologist might bandy diurnal challenges, long-standing issues, and once traumas.

Psychotherapy

It allows a psychologist to formulate an internal health opinion on the basis of psychoanalysis. A psychiatrist who conducts psychotherapy can define cases of medication. In cases of psychotherapy for alcoholism, a psychologist might help a case understand and manage their jones and stay motivated to achieve their sobriety pretensions. Psychotherapy sessions can last for several weeks or gauge numerous months.

During psychotherapy, the psychologist and case develop a relationship on the base of trust, openness, and confidentiality. Psychotherapy acts as a roadmap for clinicians. It guides them through the process of understanding their guests and developing results. There are multiple approaches to psychotherapy, similar to psychoanalysis, behavioral remedy or therapy, cognitive remedy, and integrative or holistic remedy.

Cognitive Behavioral Therapy(CBT) Cognitive Behavioral Therapy(CBT) is a proven system for easing the burdens of drunkenness. The introductory premise of CBT is the significance of relating negative studies and actions and replacing them with positive studies and actions. A CBT session will be a discussion between a case and a psychologist.

CBT is a results-acquainted approach to treatment that focuses lower on opinion and further on formative action, similar to grueling dangerous beliefs, defying fears, part-playing to ameliorate social relations, and casting strategies to stop drinking alcohol or using medicines. CBT is frequently effective with as many as five sessions.

Dialectical Behavioral Therapy(DBT) Dialectical Behavioral Therapy(DBT) is another type of substantiation-grounded talk remedy. The DBT system operates from the hypotheses that everything is connected, the world constantly changes, and contrary rudiments(thesis and antipode) may synthesize into a better element or a lesser variety.

These hypotheticals comprise the base of the philosophical system of dialectics. In practice, an individual or group DBT session will involve literacy to live in the present rather than dwelling on history, managing feelings and torture, and rehearsing honest communication. Eventually, DBT is designed to help cases find emotional balance and grasp positive change.

The system is dialectical because the guru who developed it wanted cases to be suitable to synthesize change and acceptance of history to produce a better life. Research has shown that DBT is effective for people who struggle with drunkenness and other substance abuse diseases. DBT has four main strategies that are tutored by the clinician to the customer.

• Core awareness • torture Forbearance • Interpersonal Effectiveness • Emotion Regulation

Motivational Interviewing: In counseling, motivational Interviewing (MI) is a system for encouraging a case to overcome ambivalence, set direct pretensions for tone enhancement, and stay motivated to realize them. MI is a popular fashion for treating substance abuse diseases because numerous people feel helpless against dependence and benefit from an infusion of restraint to decide to take action against it.

In a motivational interview, a therapist will encourage a case to commit to change, similar to quitting alcohol. Motivational canvassing is a detailed, customer-centered,semi-directive cerebral treatment approach that concentrates on perfecting and strengthening a customer's provocations for change. MI aims to increase a customer's perspective on the significance of the change. MI is useful for guests who are less motivated or ready for change.

The practice involves a form of probative and compassionate comforting style that rolls with resistance. MI is a brief intervention, where the counselor and customer will meet for a normal of 1 to 4 sessions. MI incorporates four introductory principles in therapy. Expressing empathy, rolling with resistance, developing tone-efficacity, and developing distinction. MI is generally enforced with other remedy modalities.

Anonymous(AA) and other 12- step programs give peer support to people quitting or cutting back on their drinking. Combined with treatment led by health professionals, collective- support groups can offer a precious added subcaste of support. A 12- Step Program supplements other forms of remedy and gives cases commodities to bandy with their psychologists.

The 12- Step approach is demonstrably effective at helping people to achieve sobriety long-term. For this reason, therapists occasionally grease the process of joining a 12- Step group for their cases and incorporate 12- Step material and their cases ' guests at meetings into their sessions.

What are 12- step programs?

Twelve-step programs give a set of principles to exercise as a way of life to manage an alcohol or medicine problem. The meetings are free of charge and are run by recovering people — rather than professional counselors who are devoted to helping themselves and others stay sober.

These programs offer people support in abstaining from alcohol and medicine use for life. Because lifelong abstinence is a significant challenge, the programs encourage people to take it " one day at a time. " Members are advised to attend regular meetings and talk about their challenges without revealing their last names(a practice known as " obscurity "). While members may have an occasional relapse or slip, where they temporarily go back to using alcohol or medicines, a 12- step program can offer retreat and access to sober support that's delicate for a floundering addict to find a way, furnishing the tools that can help arrest a relapse before it becomes a destructive curl.

Twelve-step groups also give the occasion for backing. A sponsor seen in Alcoholics Anonymous(AA) is a person with a long period of sobriety who's willing to support a recently sober person. Guarantors agree to help sponsors work through the way and to be available to help when a sponsee struggles with sobriety.

The support handed by a guarantor or sponsor while following the 12- step tone- help programs has been shown to increase the chances of abstinence. As further sober time is gained, the sponsee can also finance others, helping his or her recovery by giving back to the group.

Essential steps of the 12- step program

Step 1. Admit that you have a problem. This is an acknowledgment that you're helpless over your dependence.

Step 2. Seek help from an advanced power. At the heart of all 12- step programs is a belief that conquering dependence requires a spiritual awakening.

Step 3. Decide to turn over your life to an advanced power(still you understand the advanced power). This step involves committing to living a spiritual life rather than agreeing to join any specific religion.

Step 4. Make a moral force. Part of the recovery process involves reflecting on your history and writing a life history. The key to this process is taking responsibility for conduct and opinions.

Step 5. Entrust in someone about your once behavior. In utmost 12- step programs, the addict selects a guarantor — someone in the program who has formerly completed all the way, has a long period of sobriety and can give guidance during the recovery process.

Step 6. Work on rebuilding your character. According to the 12- step gospel, recovery entails admitting your particular failings so that you can change them.

Step 7. Ask your advanced power to remove your particular failings.

Step 8. List those whom you have harmed and come willing to make amends. While in the fray of dependence, a person frequently acts irresponsibly(for illustration, lying or stealing). To recover, addicts must admit all those whom they've hurt in history and try to make reparation.

Step 9. laboriously begin to make amends to others.

Step 10. Continue the process of taking a particular force(begun in step 4).

Step 11. Seek a near tie to your advanced power. As people in recovery develop their church, they generally use prayer and contemplation to strengthen this relationship.

Step 12. Work with others. Helping others face their addictions can boost your tone- of regard and give emotional prices.

How meetings work

Most meetings last about an hour. AA recommends that new members attend 90 meetings for the first 90 days in the program but don't pressure you to meet this thing. Members of 12- step programs are free to choose any attendance pattern that works for them. People tend to go to meetings more constantly when they're just starting the program and when they find themselves going through stressful ages. utmost members attend at least one meeting a week.

There are several types of 12- step meetings.

Open-discussion meetings. Open to addicts, their families, and anyone interested in addressing the problem of dependence. These meetings follow a set pattern. A leader describes the 12- step program and introduces one to three speakers who relate particular stories.

Unrestricted meetings. Limited to people floundering to understand their alcohol/ medicine problem and achieve sobriety, these meetings allow members to partake in their problems in trying to stay sober.

Newcomers ' meetings. In these meetings, one or further stages of the program are present to answer questions from beginners.

Step meetings. These unrestricted meetings are devoted simply to understanding the meaning of one of the 12 ways.

In addition to holding face-to-face meetings, numerous groups allow members to speak by dispatch, telephone, audio or videotape exchanges, or in online discussion forums. Group members in some programs, including AA, may make home visits to people who can't attend meetings because of an illness, injury, or disability.

Common concerns about 12- step programs

Indeed, though 12- step programs have proved to be remarkably successful for people from all walks of life, numerous people are reluctant to try one. Dubitation can also stem from a desire to avoid committing to recovery rather than from an accurate assessment of the 12- step philosophy.

Here are the common concerns: " I'm an agnostic, so the emphasis on church excludes me. " Although people in AA frequently speak of God, the program uses the term " advanced power " and gives people great freedom in interpreting it. It's described as anything outside yourself that you believe can help you to get better; it can be God, the AA fellowship, or nature if that works for you. Twelve-step programs have no ties to any systematized religion. You may define spirituality the way you wish. People of numerous beliefs belong to AA and have set up it useful to follow the way.

" I'm too shy to attend all those meetings. " numerous people at first felt this way. But the programs offer a setting that helps people ameliorate their social skills. However, you might go to meetings beforehand and offer to help set up, or stay late and help clean up, If you worry about meeting nonnatives. Having a task to negotiate can reduce social discomfort. You may also choose a meeting in a neighboring city if you don't wish to run into people you know. Eventually, battling dependence entails learning how to forge healthy connections with others. Also, keep in mind that members can choose not to partake, that is, to " pass " at any time during the meeting.

" But my real problem isn't an addiction, it's depression. " Binary diseases — a dependence plus an internal health complaint — are common among people in 12- step programs. Psychiatric treatment(for illustration, taking an antidepressant) might help your depression but may not address your dependence. frequently a combination of internal health treatment and a 12- step program is helpful. It's healthy to a flashback that indeed if dependence begins because of another cerebral issue, it becomes its primary problem that must be addressed directly.

Ways to find a 12- step group or further information.

There are some of the largest and best- known 12- step programs

Alcoholics Anonymous: The AA website includes a form to which you can enter your postal law to identify a meeting position near you. You can also shoot a communication or call AA central headquarters at1.212.870.3400.) The Online Intergroup point for AA(http//aa-intergroup.org) has information about meetings that take place by dispatch, phone, and audio or videotape exchanges.

Cocaine Anonymous: CA has information on how to find groups that can help you recover from using cocaine or any other mind-altering substance. Its online service, Cocaine Anonymous Online(http:// www.ca-online.org), has fresh programs including online meetings and Sisters in Sobriety, a dispatch support group for women.

Double Trouble in Recovery: A point for people who have both a dependence and an internal health concern. Search the point for " Double Trouble in Recovery " or DTR.

Narcotics Anonymous: NA has background information and can help you find an original support group.

12- step programs for families and musketeers of addicts Because alcohol and medicine dependence affects the entire family, there are also 12- step programs for the cousins and musketeers of addicts.

Adult Children of alcoholics: A 12- step program for people who grew up in alcoholic or else dysfunctional homes.

Al-Anon Family Groups

A tone-help program for families and friends of alcoholics, anyhow of whether the rummy is seeking help. This point also has links to Alateen, a program that helps teenagers.

Nar- Anon Family Groups A 12- step program for those affected by the dependence on someone close to them.

12- step programs for other addictions or dependencies

In recent times, 12- step programs have surfaced for a host of other dependencies including gluttony, obsessive spending or debt, sexual dependence, and gambling. These are occasionally pertained to as " process dependencies. "www.drugrehab.ca is a starting point for help in changing a 12- step behavioral dependence program. Other collective support groups include; Women for Sobriety(WFS), LifeRing, and SMART Recovery(SMART).

WFS is one of the oldest collective help druthers and the only active indispensable simply for women. WFS was innovated in 1975 as a volition to AA for women, and its development was grounded on the belief that women bear a different approach and separate meetings from men. WFS aims to support a particular commission, and its treatment/ theoretical model is grounded on a Thirteen Statement Program of positivity to encourage positive thinking, tone- regard, and emotional and spiritual growth.

There are about 62 peer-led WFS meetings nationally and 10 peer-led meetings in Canada, with roughly 4 actors per meeting; also, about 24 treatment/ recovery centers host WFS meetings led by treatment staff. Actors a) take turns reading the Thirteen Statements declarations, b) bandy content for the week, and eventually, c) partake in commodity positives that happen during the week.

LifeRing was innovated roughly 20 times after WFS, though it has roots in the aged and now substantially inactive temporal Organization for Sobriety(SOS), innovated by James Christopher in 1985. LifeRing emphasizes clergywomen in its approach, and its treatment/ theoretical model focuses on social-cognitive change strategies informed by Cognitive Behavioral remedy and Dialectical Behavioral remedy.

LifeRing encourages questions, commentary, and other feedback throughout the meeting. analogous to WFS, LifeRing's recovery thing is abstinence. There are about 163 LifeRing meetings nationally across 17 countries and fresh meetings in Canada(15), the United Kingdom(6), Ireland(9), and Sweden(5), with about 10 actors per group. Also to WFS, meetings are generally peer-led, with actors participating in response to the question, " How was your week? ".

SMART was innovated in 1994 and has roots in Rational Recovery, which is now inactive as a collective help association. (Rational Recovery, Inc. now provides information and instruction on recovery, but doesn't host groups.) SMART's " 4- Point Program " teaches tools and ways to overcome any addictive behavior, so, unlike WFS and LifeRing, isn't concentrated simply on alcohol and medicines.

SMART's program is informed by Cognitive Behavioral remedy, Rational Emotive Behavioral remedy, and Motivational improvementTherapy.Meetings generally have 3 – 25 actors per group and are led by trained facilitators including internal health/ substance abuse treatment providers, peers, or other individualities asking to help others. Facilitators need not be in recovery.

SMART meetings are more moralistic than those of WFS and LifeRing, emphasizing education on recovery tools and discussion of the material presented. The program focuses on abstinence, but individualities who aren't committed to abstinence are welcome to share and encouraged to consider how abstinence might be maintained.

CONCLUSION

Alcohol isn't an ordinary commodity. While it carries connotations of pleasure and conviviality in the minds of many, dangerous consequences of its use are different and wide. From a global perspective, to reduce the detriment caused by alcohol, programs need to take into account specific situations in different societies. Average volumes consumed and patterns of drinking are two confines of alcohol consumption that need to be considered in sweat to reduce the burden of alcohol-related problems.

Avoiding the combination of drinking and driving is an illustration of measures that can reduce the health burden of alcohol. Worldwide, alcohol takes an enormous risk on lives and communities, especially in developing countries and its donation to the overall burden of the complaint is anticipated to increase in the future.

Particularly fussing trends are the increases in the average amount of alcohol consumed per person in countries similar to China and India and the more dangerous and parlous drinking patterns among youthful people. National covering systems need to be developed to keep track of alcohol consumption and its consequences and to raise mindfulness amongst the public and policy-makers. It's over to both governments and concerned citizens to encourage debate and formulate effective public health programs that minimize the detriment caused by alcohol.